Ketogenic Diet for Beginners

Your Guide for Success

Volume 1

L.B. Daniels

Table of Contents

Chapter 1: Introduction to the Ketogenic Diet

This guidebook is an in-depth guide on everything you need to know about the ketogenic diet. You will learn absolutely everything you need to know to start a ketogenic diet successfully, use it to reach all your desired health goals, and do so with minimal efforts. If you implement these strategies, you should be able to lose about one pound of body weight each day or more. Some individuals can lose five or more pounds each day for the first three days as well as it depends on how your past dieting and eating habits were before starting to take on a ketogenic diet. This has to do with the depletion of your glycogen stores that reside in your body that attract watch, toxins, and fat.

The ketogenic diet is a sustainable diet that makes it easy to transform your health and lose weight effortlessly once you finish this book. It may seem difficult to get the hang of it at first, but soon you will find that the ketogenic diet is an easy and beneficial diet that can change your entire life. Many people who eat the ketogenic diet swear by the way it has completely changed their health, many times even eliminating major health concerns and problems. The way this diet works, you can easily reach your health goals without even having to add exercise to your schedule. However, it is recommended that you engage in at least some level of physical activity for the sake of your health. Even going for a nice 30-minute walk each morning is very beneficial when on this type of diet, but for starters you do not need to focus on that for now.

The ketogenic diet is a smart way to get healthy. All it requires is a few changes to your regular diet, and that's it. The ketogenic diet has many valuable benefits to it. You can achieve outcomes such as:

- Freedom from sugar cravings, food fixations and hypoglycemia
- Freedom from excessive hunger that a higher carbohydrate diet will trigger
- Reduced blood pressure levels
- Drop in bad (LDL) cholesterol
- A drop in your overall triglyceride levels
- Drop in blood sugar and insulin levels as well as the spikes that can occur during the day during a higher-carbohydrate diet
- Increased energy levels as you will have steady energy all day long
- Decreased joint pains and stiffness
- Eliminate brain fog and increase mental clarity
- Improved sleep patterns and decreased sleep apnea symptoms
- Effortless weight loss, especially in the first two weeks
- Relief from heartburn symptoms
- Reduced instance of gum disease and tooth decay
- Increased healthier digestion and gut health
- Better moods overall

There are many valuable benefits you can gain from a ketogenic diet. Incredibly, these benefits can be enjoyed early on in your ketogenic journey. You will find that this diet is easy to master, and that you will quickly start to see results from your efforts. Not only will you feel better overall, but your health and weight will reflect these positive health changes in your life. The ketogenic diet is a powerful, sustainable diet that can allow you to easily transform your health and maintain that transformation with minimal effort. Unlike other diets, you will not struggle to stay on track with the ketogenic diet due to much less cravings and an increased appetite suppression.

If you are ready to take the plunge and completely change your life, then you are ready for this diet! Throughout this book, you will learn about exactly what the ketogenic diet is, how you can start eating this way immediately, and the easiest way to maintain this new lifestyle. Additionally, you will learn about the many health benefits from the ketogenic diet, and how it can truly transform your life.

Please keep in mind that this book has been written for your knowledge and pleasure. Each chapter has been carefully crafted to ensure that you gain the greatest amount of information possible, while still making it easy to read and comprehend. This way, you can easily implement these new lifestyle changes into your life and feel confident and informed throughout the process. If you enjoyed this book, please look out for my other volumes of this book in the future. Enjoy the experience, and best of luck in your journey to a new you!

Chapter 2: Keto Essentials

Understanding the ketogenic diet is easy, and the way that this diet can transform your life is impressive. To truly gain all the benefits from the ketogenic diet, you must first understand exactly what it is. Understanding what the ketogenic diet entails will make it easy for you to become aware of what you will need to do to take on this diet, and master it in little to no time at all.

What "Keto" or "Ketogenic Stands for

The keto diet, or the ketogenic diet is coined based on the term "ketosis" which is the state your metabolism enters when you eat this type of diet. Ketosis means that your body is no longer consuming carbohydrates, and is instead consuming fats your body releases into your blood stream. This means that you will be gaining energy from fats and your fat reserves, instead of from carbohydrates and sugar forms like glycogen. Changing the way that you gain your energy in this manner allows for you to eat through your fat reserves and lose weight, while also staying healthy. Eating a ketogenic diet is a simple way to lose weight quickly, but stay healthy in doing so. It allows you to literally consume your fat stores for energy, and replenish your body through eating a healthy fat and nutrient rich diet that will keep you going. This type of diet is much higher in healthy dietary fat in comparison to a standard diet or even a higher carbohydrate diet. When you eat a higher-carbohydrate diet your body becomes accustomed to using sugar as a fuel instead of your body fat. Therefore, this diet is essential to losing body fat.

As you saw above, the ketogenic diet requires that you eliminate carbohydrates completely. Doing so will allow you to stop using carbohydrates for your energy, and instead start using fats for your energy. There are many carbohydrate-rich foods that you will not be able to eat when you are on the ketogenic diet. You will learn more about exactly what you can and cannot eat in later chapters, and will also get sample diet plans in the life of the ketogenic diet. You will quickly learn that it is effortless to choose meal options that are carbohydrate-free. At first, it may seem difficult. We live in a world that thrives on sugars and other carbohydrates. Soon, however, you will realize that it is extremely simple to create your own delicious meals and still eat in a way that is healthy and delicious, and that keeps you full, but doesn't have you filling up on carbohydrates that will eventually make you hungry again about an hour later. You will be able to eat in an enjoyable way *and* lose weight doing it!

Long Term Benefits

Unlike many other diets, the keto diet has many long-term benefits. There are so many valuable health transformations that you will undergo when you start to eat the keto way. Additionally, this diet is extremely easy to sustain for long periods of time, and it is healthy to do so. You do not have to worry that you are starving your body of healthy nutrients or minerals, or that you are doing harm to your body in the long run. With the ketogenic diet, you can comfortably eat this way for many years and you will not suffer because of it. If you take a daily multi-vitamin, these vitamins absorb better in a higher-fat diet as well. The vitamins A, D, E, and K require fat to be absorbed too, which are in your multi vitamin.

There are a few different styles of the ketogenic diet, each of which has its very own set of benefits. Each diet serves a unique purpose and is generally admired by a different set of people for various reasons. Below, you can explore each of the unique ketogenic diet styles:

- The Standard Keto Diet (SKD): This is the most commonly used form of the ketogenic diet, and it can be eaten by virtually anyone. It is an extremely low-carb diet that includes a moderate amount of protein and a high amount of healthy fats. The average ratio for this diet is only 5% carbohydrates, with 20% protein, and 75% fats.

- Cyclical Keto Diet (CKD): This type of diet involves eating cycles, where you alternate between low-carb and high-carb days. Generally, you will eat according to the Standard Keto Diet method for five days of the week, then eat a high-carb diet for two days. You continuously cycle between these two eating styles.

- Targeted Keto Diet (TKD): With this diet, you eat the Standard Keto Diet most of the time, but you eat high-carb meals around your workouts. This is a commonly used format for body builders and those who partake in intensive workouts.

- High-Protein Keto Diet: This diet is almost identical to the Standard Keto Diet, except that you eat a higher rate of proteins in it. You will still eat an incredibly low number of carbohydrates, around only 5% of your entire diet. But you will eat about 35% protein, and then 60% fats.

The only variations of the keto diet that has been studied extensively is the Standard Keto Diet. Virtually all studies done on the keto diet were done on those who were eating according to the SDK standards. The three alternative eating methods are more advanced and are most commonly used by high performance athletes and bodybuilders. They are generally considered to enable these individuals to have a better time building muscle, maintaining energy, and performing better overall. Still, they have not been studied as extensively as the main variation of the diet. For the average person, the Standard Keto Diet is all you will need to pay attention to. For that purpose, this book focuses solely on that variation of the diet.

Ultimately, the ketogenic diet is a low-carb, high-fat diet that is intended to eliminate fat by consuming it as an energy source. Unlike standard diets where fats are not always used effectively, the ketogenic diet eliminates carbohydrates as an energy source and uses fats to produce energy instead. As a result, you will end up losing weight and gaining several other health benefits which you will learn about soon.

Chapter 3: Ideal Keto Candidate

It is important when you are choosing to start a new diet to find one that is going to fit well with your lifestyle, including your health overall. The keto diet is a diet that is easily adapted into virtually any lifestyle, however, there are a few restrictions and considerations you should consider before taking it on yourself. Some people absolutely should not eat according to the ketogenic diet, as it can cause major health concerns that need to be looked at by a health care official. While this is rare, and it is a perfectly healthy and sustainable diet for most people, you will want to be sure that you are one of the individuals who can confidently and safely consume a ketogenic diet.

First off, you should always discuss new dietary changes with your healthcare provider. Your unique health is something that has so many variable factors that go into it, that there is simply no way this book, or any other non-qualified resource, could determine whether you are healthy enough to eat this way. While the majority of those who eat this type of diet are perfectly fine, there are a few who would not be able to eat the keto diet. In this chapter, we will discuss the guidelines and basics, but it is up to you to confirm with your doctor that this eating style will be safe for you.

You will be happy to know that if you are a healthy individual, the ketogenic diet will not harm you. This diet is completely safe if you are not suffering from any medical ailments and if you are not on any medications. Once again, if you are, you will need to confirm with your doctor that this diet is safe for you. It is extremely rare for a healthy individual to experience any form of severe or long-term side effects from this diet. While there are some side effects that are completely natural, none of them should cause you any negative health impacts.

Still, it is important to realize that there is a certain guideline for individuals who should not eat according to the ketogenic diet. If you fit the following category at all, you should not eat according to the keto diet. It is important that you understand and respect these guidelines to prevent yourself from any dangers that could occur as a result.

- If you are on medication for diabetes, you should **not** eat the ketogenic diet
- If you are a type 1 diabetic you should **not** eat the ketogenic diet
- If you are on medication for high blood pressure, you should **not** eat the ketogenic diet
- If you are breastfeeding, you should **not** eat the ketogenic diet

If you fall under any of these categories and still feel convinced that the keto diet is the way for you, then you should certainly consult your healthcare provider to further discuss this option. For the most part, if you fall into these categories, the ketogenic diet can be highly unsafe and you should never under any circumstances take on this diet without first consulting your healthcare provider. They will be able to better inform you of the potential dangers you face, should you try it. If you do not fit within these categories, then you should be fine to start eating the ketogenic diet. Many people, including body builders and high-performance athletes eat according to the keto diet and swear by it.

This diet has shown promising abilities to have significant positive impacts on their results and contribute to a major transformation on health, as well. The ketogenic diet is generally safe for anyone who is healthy to begin with, and may even be safe for some individuals who are living with certain types of diseases. Still, always ensure that your healthcare provider is on board with major dietary changes.

Chapter 4: Health Benefits

After discovering that you fit into the ideal candidate for the keto diet, you are probably curious about all the many ways that this diet can benefit your life! Of course, you saw a pretty extensive and specific list in the introduction about this, but this book isn't just about the introduction. It's about the deeper insight as to exactly how you can transform your life using these strategies that are a part of the keto diet. In this chapter, we are going to explore *exactly* what health benefits you will receive from the keto diet.

Freedom from Cravings of Sugar

As a society, we tend to consume large amounts of sugar. We eat both natural sugars and processed sugars, which can overall increase our experiences of having consistent cravings towards sweet things. Because of this, we may often find ourselves in positions where we are constantly craving sugary foods. This is not only frustrating but can be harmful, because it can lead to excessive consumptions of sugary foods that are not healthy for us. As a result, our health can shrink and suffer from our increased and excessive sugar intakes.

When you start eating according to the keto diet standards, you may feel extreme cravings towards sweet foods and sugars for the first few days. However, after some time you will notice that these cravings go away. You will no longer crave sweet foods or sugars, and eventually you will stop thinking about them altogether. Should you ever "fall off the wagon" and indulge in sugary foods, you will likely find them to taste overwhelming and perhaps even revolting. This is common for those who eat according to the ketogenic diet, and it is a form of blessing that will keep you from overindulging in sweets and treats, because you won't be indulging in them at all.

Freedom from Hypoglycemia

Our increased and excessive intakes of sugar lead to our increased resistances against sugars. Hypoglycemia can be the result of an increased intake of sugar. Essentially your body is saying "no more". When you eat according to the ketogenic diet and cut sugars out of your diet completely, you will notice that your blood sugar levels will stabilize and you will stop having symptoms associated with hypoglycemia, or type 2 diabetes.

Again, if you are an individual who lives with type 2 diabetes or who is prone to hypoglycemia, you should always check with your doctor before taking on a new diet. Although the keto diet is known to help with hypoglycemia, it is still good to keep your doctor on board with these types of changes, so no accidents or mistakes arise!

Freedom from Excessive Hunger

When you eat according to the keto diet, you will not undergo symptoms of excessive hunger like you might with other diets. That is because with the keto diet, even though you are eliminating a food group from your diet, you are not starving yourself. The keto diet works largely by eliminating an unneeded energy source and giving you the opportunity to completely nourish your body in a healthier way. When you do this, you will notice that you will not be hungry all the time, and you will feel fuller longer. The foods that you do eat when you're on the keto diet are richer and healthier, meaning they will serve your body as a fuel source for hours to come.

Reduced Blood Pressure Levels

When you eat according to the keto diet, you do not experience excessive blood pressure levels related to food intake. With a traditional or standard American diet, you may discover that you eat foods that are high in salts and sugars. This causes your blood pressure to sky rocket, especially as you receive sudden and dramatic energy bursts that only last a short period of time. Eating this way is much healthier and will eliminate the likelihood that your blood pressure will rise and fall as much, and you will eventually see that your blood pressure is likely to level out at a healthy level.

Drop in Bad Cholesterols

When you eat a keto diet, and commit to eating healthier fats, you will find that you are likely to see a major and impressive decrease in your bad cholesterol levels. Some people may not have this experience if they are not eating enough healthy fats, and are rather eating too many saturated fats. However, if you are eating according to the keto diet and you are eating healthy fats in place of saturated fats, and you are ensuring that you are taking care to keep your diet as healthy as possible, you are likely to see a drop in your bad cholesterol levels. This means that your arteries will flow easier and contributes to an overall healthier cardiovascular state.

Stabilized Blood Sugar and Insulin Levels

For those who are struggling with insulin resistance and need increased insulin sensitivity, the keto diet has been studied and shows promising results in helping treat this ailment. When you eat a high-fat keto diet, it can increase your insulin sensitivity and decrease your insulin resistance levels. In fact, in the initial study done in 2005, keto showed that it could increase insulin sensitivity by up to 75%. Since then, several studies have shown the same promising results, and several people have taken over this diet to help them increase their insulin sensitivities and feel healthier overall.

Increased Energy Levels

On a high-carbohydrate diet, you will find that you are likely to experience bursts of energy followed by bursts of exhaustion. This happens because your carbohydrates are increasing and then decreasing repeatedly. It can be very hard to maintain your carbohydrates enough to keep your energy consistent. When you eat a high-fat low-carb diet like the keto diet, though, you change your energy source to fat, instead. With your body burning fat, you will have a constant access to energy as you burn through fat reserves in your body. Since you are eating a high fat diet, you will be getting a consistent stream of fats into your body, meaning your energy levels will stay consistent and high. Those who eat according to the keto diet often report that in as little as one week their energy levels have improved significantly and that they feel much better as a result.

Decreased Joint Pain and Stiffness

Most diets these days are not healthy enough to promote healthy joints, which can lead to increased joint pain and stiffness. With a diet such as the keto diet, you eat a high-fat intake, which is important for keeping joints moving fluidly. The fat helps make the tendons and muscles move easier, and reduces instances of joint pain and stiffness. Even in individuals who struggle with arthritis have reported that the keto diet has improved their symptoms and decreased their pain and stiffness. Eating the keto diet is largely responsible for helping make the joints move easier and feel less stiff.

When you start eating the keto diet, you will likely notice improvements in as little as a couple of weeks. These improvements will continue to increase for several weeks until you are no longer experiencing such severe symptoms.

Increased Mental Clarity

Eating a diet that is rich in healthy fats directly contributes to having a healthier brain. When your brain is functioning at its best, you will have increased mental clarity. That means that you will not suffer from or struggle with the brain fog that many people claim to have, particularly in the mid-afternoon time. You will likely find that you can think clearer, recalling things easier, and have overall better brain function. This can directly translate to higher performance in life, career, and other important areas! Many people forget how important it is to eat a brain-healthy diet. When you are eating the keto way, you can feel confident that you are eating in a way that is healthy for your brain and has it functioning optimally!

Improved Sleeping Patterns

Increased and improved energy levels usually also translate to an improved sleeping pattern. Many people who eat the keto diet discover that their sleep-wake cycles regulate themselves better, and that they can sleep easier and more restfully. This is something that many people struggle with, as it can be difficult to sleep enough or restfully. When you are eating this diet, you are more likely to have a more regulated schedule which will leave you feeling even more energized and with even better mental clarity.

Weight Loss

Of course, as the title of this book suggests, the keto diet is a great way to lose weight. Many people who eat this diet lose weight quickly, and it happens in a healthy way. That means that you are not losing weight too fast for your body to maintain it, and that you are losing weight in a way that benefits your body. Because of the way the keto diet burns fat, you can rapidly burn through your fat stores. And, if you are eating a high fat diet, you will continue to burn fat and your weight will sustain itself at a healthy level. You will not need to worry about any muscle wasting or other unhealthy weight loss symptoms. Weight loss symptoms start quickly into your keto journey, with people reporting an average of about 15 pounds lost in their first two weeks on the diet.

Relief from Symptoms of Heartburn

When you eat the standard American diet, you are likely to experience symptoms of heartburn. In many people, these symptoms are severe and require treatment to maintain. Anything from over the counter medicines to prescriptions have been used to manage the symptoms of heartburn that are experienced by our nation. When you eat the keto diet, you alleviate these symptoms and reduce your likelihood of dealing with heartburn. This translates to less medicines and symptom management, as you will not have any symptoms to manage in the first place. For many people, eating this diet can completely cure heartburn associated ailments.

Reduced Instances of Gum Disease and Tooth Decay

Modern people eat extremely high levels of carbohydrates, which can directly translate to gum disease and tooth decay. Studies estimate that a shocking 47% of adults in America have some form of gum disease, which is extremely high! When you eat the keto diet, you are less likely to experience gum disease and tooth decay. The almost non-existent levels of carbohydrates in your diet means that you are not exposing your mouth to consistently and prolonged unhealthy conditions. Instead of snacking on candies, chips, crackers, or other carbohydrate-rich foods, you will be snacking on healthier food choices such as vegetables. Even better, if you snack on harder vegetables like carrots, you will further reduce your likelihood of experiencing gum disease or tooth decay.

Increased Healthy Digestion and Gut Health

Eating a better diet that is nutrient-rich and full of healthy macros means that you're going to experience better gut health overall. Your body will have an easier time digesting food as you will not be eating any processed foods, and as a result your gut health will be healthier overall. Just like your symptoms of heartburn will reduce, so too will your symptoms of any other digestion-related ailments. You will quickly see an improvement in these conditions and will find that you have an easier time breaking down foods, absorbing the healthy nutrients from them, and passing them through your system.

A combination of these healthy transformations in your life are what contribute to your better overall mood. When you have a healthier brain and a system that is functioning better, you are more likely to experience better moods overall. Your increased energy and better sleeping patterns will assist with this, too.

You will probably start noticing that you are happier more often, and that you are easily able to cope with stress and other overwhelming emotions. As you can see, there is an incredible number of benefits that comes from eating the keto diet. When you eat this high-fat low-carb diet, you will be more likely to experience better health inside and out. Your body will function better, your brain will be healthier, you will lose extra weight, and you will be able to quite literally watch your health and body transform.

Additionally, you will experience a better mood overall, as well as higher energy levels and more restful sleep. The longer you eat the keto way, the more you will reap in the benefits that this diet offers. This diet is one of the healthiest and most sustainable diets you could choose to undertake.

Chapter 6: Eating the Keto Way

The ketogenic diet is, as you've read already, a high-fat low-carb diet that relies on the state of ketosis to work. As we mentioned back in chapter one, this book is aimed to guide you through eating the Standard Keto Diet (SKD), so this section is going to teach you exactly how you can eat according to those standards. If you choose to eat according to a different method of the keto diet, most the information will stay the same. The only difference will be how much carbs you eat, and when you will eat them. As a beginner, it's a good idea to transition into the keto diet faster than you may with others. Rather than gradually eliminating carbohydrates, you should consider cutting them out altogether. Or, cutting out the extremely unhealthy ones first, and then about a week or two later, cutting out the rest. The sooner you get the carbohydrates out of your diet, the sooner you can work on kicking your cravings towards them and fully embracing the keto diet lifestyle.

The easiest way to get into ketosis is to make sure that you are eating at least less than 50 grams of carbs every single day. Ideally, you want to be under 20 grams. The less carbs you are eating, the better. You will need to completely cut out and avoid sugary foods, as well as starchy foods. You should not be eating obvious things like candies, chocolate bars, baked goods, and other treats that have sugar in them.

Additionally, you should not be eating starchy goods such as bread, pasta, and potatoes. These are rich in carbohydrates, and will keep your body out of the state of ketosis. To effectively eat this diet and gain benefits from it, you will need to ensure that you are entering the state of ketosis, and maintaining it. You do this by eliminating the carbohydrates from your diet.

A general guideline for your food intake is to eat less than 5-10% of carbohydrates every day, about 15-25% protein, with the lower end being the most effective, and about 70% or more of healthy fats. You want to make sure that you really put an emphasis on eating healthy fats, and that you aren't consuming an excessive amount of saturated fats or other unhealthy fats. These are the types that can contribute to higher cholesterol. You want to make sure that you aren't doing that. Below is a more in-depth list of what you can eat and what you should avoid. It may seem difficult at first, but once you realize what is carbohydrate-rich, you will have an easy time remembering and avoiding it.

Remember, you will want to make sure that you are also monitoring your drinks. Some drinks, such as alcohol and juices, are going to be rich in carbohydrates. You will want to avoid these, as these will also sabotage your ketosis. Ideally, you should not be drinking any of these things. If you do, you will not be in a state of ketosis and you will not be gaining the benefits of the ketogenic diet. You don't want to make the mistake of altering your entire eating habits, and drinking the same way as you always have as this will sabotage all your hard effort that you have put in to eating a healthier diet! For that reason, drinks are also included on the What Not to Eat and What to Eat lists.

Eat This	Not This
Beef	Fruit
Pork	Potatoes
Lamb	Pasta
Game	Beer
Poultry	Rice
Fish and Shellfish	Bread
Eggs	Donuts
Natural Fat and High Fat Sauces	Chocolate
Green vegetables	Candy
Dairy Products	Soda
Nuts	Juice
Berries	Alcohol

Water	Processed Foods (EVEN "keto friendly" ones should be avoided)
Tea and Coffee	**SOMETIMES you can drink regular red wine, dry white wine, whisky, brandy, vodka, and cocktails without sugar**

It is very important that you avoid foods that are labelled as "ketogenic friendly" as many of these will not actually be ketogenic friendly. Sadly, they can falsely label their products and you will find that they are often loaded with products that are not keto friendly and therefore will take you out of ketosis. Additionally, you can occasionally indulge in alcohols and dark chocolate, if you ensure you aren't doing it on a regular basis.

It may feel difficult at first to stick to the keto diet when you see that all the convenient foods are cut out of your list. You will not want to eat these foods, as many of them contain sugars as a preservative, and this will take you out of ketosis. If you are someone who enjoys convenient meals, you can still enjoy a convenient meal on the keto diet. A great way to do this is to meal prep your food a few days in advance, and simply pop them in the microwave or in a pan on the stove top to reheat them. This allows you to save yourself from having to cook during times that may be busy, but also gives you the ability to stay within' your keto diet.

It also may seem as though you are cutting a lot of food out of your diet. You are not. You are still able to eat several whole and nutritional foods. You are only cutting out ones that are high in sugars or carbohydrates, as these will keep you from entering ketosis and will sabotage your ability to gain any of the benefits from the keto diet, since you won't be eating true to it.

Again, it may seem difficult to cut these foods out at first, but once you become used to it, you won't even miss them. As a society, we tend to crave sweet and sugary foods a lot more than we need them. In fact, we don't need them at all. We like them, however, because they are easy to make and they taste good. It may be hard to let go of your favorites, but in time you will find new favorites.

If you are really struggling to let go of some of your higher carb foods, a good idea is to spend some time before you embark on your full keto diet discovering new recipes. This will give you a chance to explore and create new favorites, without feeling pressured to. Or, if you're someone who likes to jump in feet first, you can gather as many delicious ingredients from your grocery store as possible and spend the entire first week eating brand new meals and finding out what your new favorites are.

You may be surprised to learn that just because you are on a keto diet doesn't mean you can't enjoy treats and snacks. In fact, there are copious amounts of keto friendly dessert recipes and treat recipes available these days. That is one of the great benefits of having a sustainable diet that people can eat for long periods of time: new recipes are always coming to the surface, and they taste good, too! If you are someone who loves a good dessert, you can usually discover an easy and tasty recipe for a tasty treat quickly online or in a keto friendly recipe book.

If you are still struggling to figure out exactly what you are going to eat daily, below you will find a meal plan that will give you an idea as to what you could eat over a period of five days on the keto diet. You will notice that these foods are high in fats, and very low in carbohydrates, and lower in proteins. These meals are easy to make, and you can modify them in any way you desire. Unlike many other diets, you won't really need a recipe book to get started on the keto diet, as most meals contain whole-food ingredients. That makes it easier for you to start eating this way, right away. As well as to make your desired modifications any time you want!

Five Day Meal Plan

Here is a five-day meal plan of what people eat on a keto diet. You will see that it is high fat, medium protein and low carb. This diet will assist you in reaching a state of ketosis, which means that you will be eating the right way to reap in the full benefits of the keto diet.

Day 1:

Breakfast: Two eggs, scrambled with goat cheese and seasoned with herbs. Side of bacon, and a cup of coffee.

Lunch: Yogurt, cheese slices, a cup of nuts and seeds, sugar-free peanut butter on celery sticks.

Dinner: Grilled salmon topped with homemade creamy lemon sauce with a side of keto-friendly vegetables and high-fat dip.

Dessert: A slice of dark chocolate

Day 2:

Breakfast: One cup of cottage cheese with cinnamon and pecan nuts, milk to drink.

Lunch: A salad topped with grilled chicken and sesame seeds, with a high-fat low-carb dressing.

Dinner: Steak topped with mushrooms and a small amount of tomatoes, with a side of Brussel sprouts.

Day 3:

Breakfast: Three sausage patties, a cup of steamed spinach

Lunch: Lettuce wrap stuffed with ground beef, cheese, and roasted vegetables

Dinner: Stir fry with turkey

Day 4:

Breakfast: Bacon with two hard boiled eggs and a small salad with sugar free dressing

Lunch: Pepperoni, celery sticks with cheese, handful of nuts and seeds.

Dinner: Grilled chicken with roasted vegetables and a glass of full-fat milk

Dessert: 2-3 strawberries with cream and a few tablespoons of almond butter

Day 5:

Breakfast: Steak and eggs with a few handfuls of spinach and sweet onions sautéed

Lunch: Salad with full-fat dressing with pepperoni on the side

Dinner: Grilled white fish with two poached eggs as well as two cups of steamed broccoli

As you can see, living the keto lifestyle is tasty, fun, and memorable. You can swap out certain ingredients for others and remain successful in your endeavors as well. Just remember to stay away from carbohydrates and you are on your way to a new you!

Chapter 7: Exercise is Not Required to Lose Weight

Exercise and working out is important, but not nearly as important as the food you eat, what type of food you eat, but most importantly, the calories in those foods you eat, that regulate your body mass. If you force your body to burn calories then when you are at rest you may burn less calories to a certain degree. Athletes have such low heart rates when at rest because when they burn many calories during the day they have ended up training their body to burn less calories when they aren't exercising. The human body has a way of balancing itself out. If you are cold, your body heat turns up, if you are hot, you sweat to cool down. If you force your body to burn calories, you will train your body to burn calories less in other ways.

One way an individual may believe exercise burns calories is that just having an exercise routine causes a person to clean up their food intake. Also, individuals that tend to exercise a lot typically use a supplement that contains caffeine (even if it is just coffee), which suppresses appetite and causes you to fidget more and move more altogether. Even if the body tries to regulate how many calories it wants to burn, if you exercise a lot, you will burn more calories than your body can down regulate during the other parts of the day.

One way for your body to down-regulate its caloric burning properties if you do a lot of cardiovascular activities is to burn off some muscle, so you look less lean and more like a marathon runner. Have you ever seen a marathon runner? They are very slim and frail looking because they have burned off a lot of their muscles from all the cardiovascular exercise they are doing to prepare for their marathons. Look at a sprinter, they train with sprints for their cardio, and they also take on resistance training for their bursts of speed. Marathon runners don't generally do resistance training as they need to be as light as possible.

Exercise is great, but it is something you add on to a healthy eating plan to maximize your weight loss. If you were to compare the two types of exercise, cardiovascular exercise (cardio), or resistance training (lifting weight and the such), you may want to look to resistance training, as you build muscle and tone your body in addition to burning calories. Cardio just aims to burn calories and your body will build a tolerance to that, but the tolerance your body creates to resistance training is strength, more muscle and tone, which burns more calories when at rest than cardio.

Exercise is good for health, but don't do too much. Moderation is the key, and this goes with cardio and resistance training and eating healthy. You need to create a balance. Weight gain is mostly from two things: Too many calories from foods you eat during the day followed by too much inactivity. Some individuals may thing their lack of activity is what caused their weight gain, but it's not so true in the way that they think. It isn't because you are burning less calories during the day, it is because inactivity causes boredom and boredom causes you to want to eat more. We will go through this in further chapters.

Calories are the form of energy we get out of food. If you take a "calorimeter", which is a certain heating device, and toss various foods in it, you get a certain number of calories burnt out of it. Toss in some steak, calories. Toss in some bread, calories. Toss in some broccoli, calories. Toss in the insides of a tree, you get calories. For the tree, yes, in Papua New Guinea they eat the inside of trees, and they have generally the same caloric value as potatoes. Hell, let's go ahead and toss in Gasoline into that calorimeter (Don't drink gasoline, please!), and you get calories. Okay, so gasoline makes a car run, right? Well it's the calories that do it. It's the heat that is generated that does it. For example, a calorie is the energy needed to increase the temperature of a given mass of water by 1 degrees Celsius.

Let's view the human body as a machine for a second. It takes a lot of food each day to run, and specific foods give off certain kinds of macronutrients and micronutrients, sure. But in the end of all things, what makes the human body run is Calories. The average man, regardless of bodyweight to an extent, needs about 2700 calories a day to stay the same weight. If this man is 150 pounds, or 300 pounds, about 2700 calories will keep him that weight. A woman needs about 2100 calories per day to maintain any weight she is at as well under the same circumstances.

Exercise increases how many calories you burn, in which makes you lose weight, but as stated in previous chapters, your body will fight back to balance out your expenditure. Your body has one job, and one job only: to keep you alive. If you stress it, it will find a way to cope with that stress and you become stronger. If a marathon runner runs many hours a day, the body will view that as stress and make it easier to run for hours a day, be it a lower heart rate, less muscle mass, and of course less body fat.

Calories are the units of energy your body uses to maintain your body through all bodily processes during the day. That is over-simplifying it because when you say a man burns about 2700 calories a day and a woman burns about 2100 calories a day, this is taking in all different processes that are going on under the hood, so to speak.

For the three macro-nutrients: Protein, Carbohydrates, and Fat, they all have various modes of action. When your body burns them, they give off a certain caloric value: Protein and Carbohydrates burn at about 4 calories for each gram, and fat burns at about 9 calories per gram. It may look simple to remove fat from your diet to lose weight, but luckily it makes you feel fuller than carbohydrates and protein to a certain degree.

Carbohydrates are burned and turned into glucose to keep your blood sugar (energy) regulated. Your body can only have about one teaspoon of glucose in your bloodstream at one time or you will die, so your body uses the hormones insulin and glucagon to keep it going and coming. Protein and Dietary fat is used for various hormone production. Protein can turn into glucose when burned as well, but the body does not prefer it, and dietary fat can be used as energy as ketones when your blood sugar is low as well.

Chapter 9: How Your Body Burns Fat

For basic measures, a pound of fat when burned by the human body, is about 3500 calories. If a man (burning 2700 calories a day), eats about 2200 calories, he will have burned about 500 more than he ate, which in turn the body required from his body fat, so he would be at a "deficit" for the day of about -500. If this man did this for 7 days straight, he would be at a deficit of about 3500 calories, and in return, he would have burned about 1 pound of fat from his body in various locations. That's all. For the same thing to happen for a woman that burns about 2100 calories a day, a woman would just need to eat 1600 calories. Women burn about 2100 calories per day because of less muscle mass, but luckily, they have less of an appetite to compensate so to speak.

If a person, regardless of their current bodyweight, eats roughly 500 calories more than they burn each day, and does this for about 7 days, they will gain one pound of fat somewhere on their body in various locations. Do this for 52 weeks or one year, and there is your 50+ pound weight gain that just snuck up on you. This is exactly how body weight loss and gain happens. You put food in, and calories come out.

Chapter 10: Feeling Full and Feeling Hungry

For general information, the hormone that tells you to stop eating is called leptin. The other hormone that tells you to eat is ghrelin. If you eat foods with high sugar content, your blood sugar will spike, and your pancreas will release a hormone called insulin, and this will drive your blood sugar back down. But, this also means you will have lower blood sugar now, so you will feel weak and low on energy and hungry again, so your body will release ghrelin to get you to eat again.

Ever eat Chinese food? Have you ever felt hungry again an hour or so later? This is exactly that, but it also works with high sugar or high carbohydrate foods. Therefore, a lower carbohydrate diet may be good for you, but it doesn't mean it's the best solution, it just means watch out for foods that spike your blood sugar too high, like rice, pasta, potatoes, sugar, candy and sodas.

What this all means is that individuals may have trouble with their appetites, and their body's mechanisms will make them eat depending on the foods they eat, but when it comes down to it, it still matters about calories. Yes, certain eating patterns and selections of food have certain amounts of calories, but these calories may be adjusting your leptin and ghrelin signals to make you eat irregularly. If you ignored these signals and ate a specific number of calories each day to lose weight, you would succeed.

A lot of diets try to get around this and tell you to eat certain types of foods in hopes that this signaling puts you in a caloric deficit without getting too complex about things. It works for some people, and it doesn't work for some people. It honestly really depends. If you don't like to eat too much and go on an Atkins style diet, you may lose weight because not only does protein and dietary fat cause your appetite to be suppressed, you don't like eating that way anyway. But losing weight isn't about dieting and getting off diets back and forth, that can't be healthy mentally and physically.

So, if you are put on an Atkins style diet, lose some weight, and return to your normal eating, you will gain the weight back because you did not make any lasting changes. A lasting change to something like that would be to incorporate meat into your normal food schedules if you didn't eat that much meat before, so that may help with suppressing your appetite.

There are individuals that have lost weight on a 'Twinkie' style diet, by just eating about 1800 calories a day and proceed about two pounds of fat loss each week until they decided to return to normal eating. That is interesting, because eating only addicting foods can be a challenge, but they did it. Eating only junk food though also means you will not be getting any vitamins or minerals to keep you healthy, so I hope those individuals also took a multi vitamin at the very least.

Chapter 11: Journaling for Success

Sometimes, losing weight could be as simple as looking at what you are eating. It is very easy to just wake up, eat whatever you see in the kitchen or whatever is nearby or looks good on the way to work. It's easy to grab a snack or two at work and drop by a fast food restaurant on the way home after it all. Sometimes foods don't look so fattening or high in calories, so it is easy to live each day thinking everything is okay, when the weight is creeping up.

What this means is, if you do anything to start any program, to ease into it, you may want to take a week or two and just write down everything you are eating. Just this might take care of things. There is such a thing in psychology of cash versus credit cards, it is much easier to swipe your credit card and forget you bought that item versus handing out actual cash, your brain registers it differently, so with that said, mindlessly eating food versus just writing it down may reduce your food consumption to the point that your weight reduces enough to make you happy to start.

If after a week or two things are not taking care of themselves, then look at how you are recording your food consumption. Writing "a slice of pizza" is different than saying you had "a large slice of meat lover's pizza" from your favorite restaurant that loves to top off your pizzas with ingredients. For general knowledge, if you only drink diet soda, they are useful because they have no calories, but the artificial sweeteners can increase appetite, so be weary.

Chapter 12: Weigh yourself each week

A lot of individuals take on a weight loss journey, but weigh themselves many times a day or at times that are not consistent. It is very easy to weight yourself in the morning and by the time you go to sleep to weight yourself and wonder where many pounds came from. Of course, food has weight, but how does this change from the time you fall asleep and wake up? Water. As you sleep, your body will expel water at a very slow rate as well as when you wake up you will typically use the restroom, so that extra weight goes away.

Some individuals also choose to weigh each day, or every couple day, being very inconsistent, which makes one bad day make someone think that their weight loss efforts are not working. For example, even if you did not eat too much, if you ate fast food or take out one night, that type of food may be high in carbohydrates and very high in sodium, which binds to water that you ingest for a few days, so the next day you may appear to have gained body fat, when it was just water.

From here, just take note to weigh yourself once a week under the same conditions. For example, I like to weigh myself on Saturday morning as soon as I wake up, right after using the restroom and brushing my teeth. I do this for 4 weeks and take note to my weight as it changes. If my weight stays the same each week or increases, then I know I need to pull back my food intake and/or calories.

Bonus 1: Weight Loss Template

Journaling your food intake is a must when it comes to weight loss. One of the major reasons weight gain slowly creeps up on an individual is that they are not paying attention to what they are eating and accidently overconsume enough to cause weight gain. It is very easy to mindlessly consume food when you have a busy, hectic and on the go schedule, but that makes weight gain easy. It is time to start journaling your food intake.

If you purchased the paperback version of this book, below is a 2-week weight loss template that you should fill out each day. As you fill out the template with what you ate and drank each day, on day 7 and 14, weigh yourself and record your bodyweight. This will tell you if you are making any progress with your eating plan. You can weigh yourself more frequently, but it is advised to do it every seven days for more accurate results.

After you complete the fourteen-day weight loss template, I have also created an advanced weight loss template that will help you understand your weight loss and/or weight stall if you still are stalling. Keep it up and you will find losing weight is simple and fun! Patience is the best variable when it comes to weight loss.

Weight Loss Template

Day 1   Weight ______

Directions:

Write your food and drink intake as accurately as you can. Each day you will get better at doing so.

Weight Loss Template

Day 2

Directions:

Write your food and drink intake as accurately as you can. Each day you will get better at doing so.

Weight Loss Template

Day 3

Directions:

Write your food and drink intake as accurately as you can. Each day you will get better at doing so.

Weight Loss Template

Day 4

Directions:

Write your food and drink intake as accurately as you can. Each day you will get better at doing so.

Weight Loss Template

Day 5

Directions:

Write your food and drink intake as accurately as you can. Each day you will get better at doing so.

Weight Loss Template

Day 6

Directions:

Write your food and drink intake as accurately as you can. Each day you will get better at doing so.

Weight Loss Template

Day 7   **Weight** _______

Directions:

Write your food and drink intake as accurately as you can. Each day you will get better at doing so.

____

____

____

____

____

____

____

____

____

____

____

____

____

____

____

____

____

____

____

____

____

____

Weight Loss Template

Day 8

Directions:

Write your food and drink intake as accurately as you can. Each day you will get better at doing so.

Weight Loss Template

Day 9

Directions:

Write your food and drink intake as accurately as you can. Each day you will get better at doing so.

Weight Loss Template

Day 10

Directions:

Write your food and drink intake as accurately as you can. Each day you will get better at doing so.

Weight Loss Template

Day 11

Directions:

Write your food and drink intake as accurately as you can. Each day you will get better at doing so.

Weight Loss Template

Day 12

Directions:

Write your food and drink intake as accurately as you can. Each day you will get better at doing so.

Weight Loss Template

Day 13

Directions:

Write your food and drink intake as accurately as you can. Each day you will get better at doing so.

Weight Loss Template

Day 14   **Weight** ______

Directions:

Write your food and drink intake as accurately as you can. Each day you will get better at doing so.

Bonus 2: Advanced Weight Loss Template

Congratulations on reaching day 14 on the weight loss template! How was journaling your food intake? Did your weight change? Let's go into some details about weight loss that will help you in further progress or help you get over a hurdle. Weight loss is simple, but it also can be complicated if you let it be.

All food is made up of three macronutrients: Protein, Carbohydrates, and Dietary Fat. Protein and Carbohydrates have a caloric value of 4 calories per gram, and dietary fat has a caloric value of 9 calories per gram.

What is a calorie you say? It is the type of energy your body extracts out of the food you eat. The average man needs 2700 calories each day to maintain his weight, and the average woman requires 2100 calories per day.

A pound of fat on the human body has a value of 3500 calories. For example, as a woman, if you ate 1600 calories each day, you would technically be in a deficit of 500 calories for that day. If you did this for one week, you would lose exactly one pound of fat and additionally, your body would purge some toxins from your body fat as well.

In addition to journaling your food intake, please record the calories in these foods you are eating. If there are no nutrition facts label on the products you are eating, do a google search on what you ate and there should be a website that has calculated it for you.

Advanced Weight Loss Template

Day 1   Weight ______

Directions:

Write your food and drink intake as accurately as you can. Write the calories to the right.

____   ______

____   ______

____   ______

____   ______

____   ______

____   ______

____   ______

____   ______

____   ______

____   ______

____   ______

____   ______

____   ______

Total ______

Advanced Weight Loss Template

Day 2

Directions:

Write your food and drink intake as accurately as you can. Write the calories to the right.

____ ________

____ ________

____ ________

____ ________

____ ________

____ ________

____ ________

____ ________

____ ________

____ ________

____ ________

____ ________

____ ________

Total ________

Advanced Weight Loss Template

Day 3

Directions:

Write your food and drink intake as accurately as you can. Write the calories to the right.

____ ______

____ ______

____ ______

____ ______

____ ______

____ ______

____ ______

____ ______

____ ______

____ ______

____ ______

____ ______

____ ______

Total ______

Advanced Weight Loss Template

Day 4

Directions:

Write your food and drink intake as accurately as you can. Write the calories to the right.

____   _______

____   _______

____   _______

____   _______

____   _______

____   _______

____   _______

____   _______

____   _______

____   _______

____   _______

____   _______

____   _______

Total   _______

Advanced Weight Loss Template

Day 5

Directions:

Write your food and drink intake as accurately as you can. Write the calories to the right.

_______________________________________ _______

_______________________________________ _______

_______________________________________ _______

_______________________________________ _______

_______________________________________ _______

_______________________________________ _______

_______________________________________ _______

_______________________________________ _______

_______________________________________ _______

_______________________________________ _______

_______________________________________ _______

_______________________________________ _______

Total _______

Advanced Weight Loss Template

Day 6

Directions:

Write your food and drink intake as accurately as you can. Write the calories to the right.

Total ______

Advanced Weight Loss Template

Day 7   Weight ______

Directions:

Write your food and drink intake as accurately as you can. Write the calories to the right.

________________________________   ______

________________________________   ______

________________________________   ______

________________________________   ______

________________________________   ______

________________________________   ______

________________________________   ______

________________________________   ______

________________________________   ______

________________________________   ______

________________________________   ______

________________________________   ______

________________________________   ______

Total   ______

Advanced Weight Loss Template

Day 8

Directions:

Write your food and drink intake as accurately as you can. Write the calories to the right.

_______________________________________   _______

_______________________________________   _______

_______________________________________   _______

_______________________________________   _______

_______________________________________   _______

_______________________________________   _______

_______________________________________   _______

_______________________________________   _______

_______________________________________   _______

_______________________________________   _______

_______________________________________   _______

_______________________________________   _______

_______________________________________   _______

Total   _______

Advanced Weight Loss Template

Day 9

Directions:

Write your food and drink intake as accurately as you can. Write the calories to the right.

_______________________________________ _______

_______________________________________ _______

_______________________________________ _______

_______________________________________ _______

_______________________________________ _______

_______________________________________ _______

_______________________________________ _______

_______________________________________ _______

_______________________________________ _______

_______________________________________ _______

_______________________________________ _______

_______________________________________ _______

_______________________________________ _______

Total _______

Advanced Weight Loss Template

Day 10

Directions:

Write your food and drink intake as accurately as you can. Write the calories to the right.

_______________________________________ ______

_______________________________________ ______

_______________________________________ ______

_______________________________________ ______

_______________________________________ ______

_______________________________________ ______

_______________________________________ ______

_______________________________________ ______

_______________________________________ ______

_______________________________________ ______

_______________________________________ ______

_______________________________________ ______

_______________________________________ ______

Total ______

Advanced Weight Loss Template

Day 11

Directions:

Write your food and drink intake as accurately as you can. Write the calories to the right.

____ ______

____ ______

____ ______

____ ______

____ ______

____ ______

____ ______

____ ______

____ ______

____ ______

____ ______

____ ______

____ ______

Total ______

Advanced Weight Loss Template

Day 12

Directions:

Write your food and drink intake as accurately as you can. Write the calories to the right.

Total ______

Advanced Weight Loss Template

Day 13

Directions:

Write your food and drink intake as accurately as you can. Write the calories to the right.

Total ______

Advanced Weight Loss Template

Day 14   Weight ______

Directions:

Write your food and drink intake as accurately as you can. Write the calories to the right.

___________________________________   _____

___________________________________   _____

___________________________________   _____

___________________________________   _____

___________________________________   _____

___________________________________   _____

___________________________________   _____

___________________________________   _____

___________________________________   _____

___________________________________   _____

___________________________________   _____

___________________________________   _____

___________________________________   _____

                                    Total   _____

Conclusion

Weight loss is a life-long journey, but it does not have to be painful. Individuals are so busy with their lives that they end up eating on the go, and just enjoying life a little too much, but this in turn creates a problem, a weight problem. Think of it this way, if you went to purchase something, how would you feel if you swiped a credit card, grabbed the receipt, tossed it into the trash and went on with your business? Compare to that to seeing the price tag of the items you bought and had to physically give cash for the items you purchased. After that, receive the receipt and look at what you purchased? Which scenario would help you regulate your costs and reduce the chance you would go into debt?

This applies to weight loss the same way but in reverse, instead of going into debt, you gain weight. It's that simple, but also complex if you are used to eating anything when you have the time or when you have a craving and such.

I hope you enjoyed this book and hope you become successful in your weight loss endeavors. You can do it! I believe in you.

L.B. Daniels